I0429137

Naturally Healthy and Happy

My Simple Guide to Living a Holistic Lifestyle

DEDICATION

Firstly, I dedicate this book to Ben P. He has no idea how many people he has helped by helping us build our dream at FFC. Thank you from me, and all the FFC folks!

And mostly, I dedicate this book to my husband Damon who let me use his real name and stories from our real life. Thanks for keeping me laughing and for you love and encouragement. P.S. All my love.

DISCLAIMER

For more information please contact:

Laurel@floridafitnesscoaches.com

TABLE OF CONTENTS

INTRODUCTION – WHO AM I AND WHY DID I WRITE THIS BOOK?

Speaking as a child of the 70s/80s I can tell you I am writing this book to offset my own personal carbon footprint. You see, I believe that my aqua-net usage in the 80s may be partly responsible for the hole in the ozone.

I was born in Waterville, Maine, in 1972. I grew up on Lucky Charms, whole milk and Devil Dogs. I remember the first TV remote control that was wired to our TV set, and MTV's debut. I did aerobics in front of the TV with my babysitter. In high school I ate chocolate chip ice cream sandwiches and drank chocolate milk everyday. I hated gym class and sports and was generally non-athletic, and I did not have the heart of a warrior at all.

In college in the 90s I met my husband, Damon. He was a bodybuilder athlete and pretty much my polar opposite. I was 98lbs soaking wet, and he will tell you that I could not ride the stationary bicycle at the gym he worked at for more than 3 minutes! I had no muscle. I ate chocolate glazed donuts and drank Dunkin Donuts coffee loaded up with plenty of Equal every day. He was shocked and horrified when I told him I put whole milk on my cereal. Welcome to the 90s, the beginning of the fat-free craze.

When I met him I was introduced to whey protein. We made everything from Diet Fuel. I was also introduced to step aerobics and lifting weights. We ate fat-free Entenmann's cakes and had only skim milk in our house. Damon's entire family was into health and fitness; his parents started a gym in their community and his little sister placed 3rd in a bodybuilding show when she was 16, very impressive. Remember, I never lifted weights, I was not competitive in sports and my entire diet revolved around sugar. However, thus began my journey into the realm of health and fitness and the land of chicken and rice.

These people impressed me, and I wanted to be strong and healthy. Back then Damon's parents looked like they were barely 30 years old, and today they are well into their 60s and they definitely hold the standard for how strong and healthy I want to be when I grow up!

Damon and I moved out of Maine to sunny Florida in 2002. He was working for a well-known nutrition and supplement company and had tripled his territory up north, so after we had taken a few trips to Florida to visit his folks we thought, "Why wait until we retire to not live in miserable cold?" and he asked for a transfer.

That's when I began personal training. I had been working as an operations manager for a World Gym up north, and I had also been working with Damon as my trainer and personal fitness professional when I decided to get my NASM (National Academy of Sports Medicine) certification. Damon is another inspiration and reason why I do what I do. There is no one I look up to more in this industry than him. He reads and absorbs everything that's new and exciting in the field. He has a real passion for fitness and learning and helping people. Anyway, it was a great job as it was flexible and we had a young son, so it allowed me to be home before and after school. There were enough people down here that were retired and could work within my schedule. We live in Naples, Florida, the land of the retired. So I worked with a lot of older people, and I really, truly enjoyed it. I trained in a commercial gym down here and in homes until one of my clients offered to build me a gym...yeah I know, long story but it ends with a murder. No, just kidding, it ends with us being where we are today: owning our own gym, Florida Fitness Coaches.

As a trainer, the majority of the people I have worked with over the years have wanted to lose weight and improve their everyday lives. I was schooled by my certifying body on the correct ways to improve balance and core stabilization and I brought this to my people. In the early 2000s there weren't many people who had done more at the gym than sit on some contraption and move the weight bars up and down ten times/repeat for every single other machine in the place. I would look around at other trainers ogling girls or checking their phones as their clients sat on machines and struggled through bad form and horrible programming. I wondered if they had ever even consulted with their clients as to what THEIR goals are, or just inflicted their own ideas about what they need onto them. Come to think of it, I never EVER saw another trainer in that big gym do an assessment, either movement or goal assessment or otherwise. A lot of those clients continued to look the same day in and day out, no matter how many times they came to the gym and no matter how much money they paid, including some of my own clients I am ashamed to say. Back then I always wondered why I had to work out to stay in shape, and these guys were enormous but I had never seen them lift a weight. Oh yeah, steroids.

Remember what I said about who I mostly trained down here in southwest Florida: mostly people over 50, A LOT of them with injuries, artificial knees, surgeries and a long list of medications. The cool thing is these people, no matter how old or no matter what they had been through, knew the importance of exercise. A lot of these people were trying not only to move better but also lose weight. Hey, who doesn't want to be sexy for life?

Back in those days we taught the energy in/energy out mantra. You must eat less than you move to lose weight. I can remember telling people they could eat 1200 calories of Twinkies and lose weight, that it didn't matter what you ate as long as they ate less than they burned. Ah yes, the LAW of thermodynamics. I talked about that law a lot. Anyway, I never told people to actually eat only Twinkies, I probably could have gotten rich if I published it then; I can see it now, "Body BY Twinkies".

As time progressed, Damon and I could both see a difference in the client of the millennium and the client of 10 years before. People were fatter and sicker than they had previously been, and the usual energy in energy out tactics began to not be as effective. I actually began to think that the Twinkies, soda and Oreos of today had changed a lot from when I was packing them for my lunch in junior high school.

I was even gaining weight though my workouts were the same and our diet had not changed. I began to really notice after my sandwich of whole wheat bread and turkey breast or even PB&J that I absolutely HAD to lay my head down. I could not make it through the afternoon without a little nap. Prior to me learning anything about gluten I knew I had to give that up. I started coaching people to eat less out of a box, like put the Wheat Thins down man, because before you even know what happened, you are looking at the bottom of the box, and you still don't feel full!

The business had changed from taking people through workouts (good balanced workouts) to dealing with problems like the ones I was having: weight gain and acne. People had begun to take a whole host of new drugs; I have trained so many men with prostate cancer it doesn't even phase me now. I have heard the gory details of some of the most gory and masochistic procedures in the medical field.

The more I was struggling with my health, and the more I would hear about my clients struggling with their health, and the grosser the surgery and the longer the list of side effects from the medications people would rattle off, the more I knew I needed to get a handle on my health, and help people find answers and take control of their own health.

I am not even going to get on my soapbox about healthcare. All I can say is each day the government tries to get more involved in our own personal family business, the more we must take responsibility for our own lives and choices.

In 2012 I took a course in Holistic Lifestyle Coaching with Paul Chek. This course introduced me to a whole new world of coaching and new methods of helping people reach their goals and get healthier and take charge! It helped me understand why I was feeling so lousy physically and how to change my ways. I have since taken more courses in Holistic Lifestyle Coaching and began to coach our training clients at FFC on how to live in optimal health!

Anyway, I am telling you all of this so you know where I am coming from for the rest of this story. I don't really consider this a how-to book: it's not a guide to get ripped in 4 minutes a day or a book telling you how to live. This is simply a collection of my musings, as well as things I have done that have worked and not worked for me. It's a collection of the research I have done and the classes I have taken, it is my own personal road to health thus far. I don't believe in perfection or perfect balance. I believe in being educated and making good informed choices. Our ideas about health and fitness have changed over the years as you can hopefully already tell. I don't think that means we were wrong, I think that means we have evolved and changed with the times. We have learned so much about the body and exercise and nutrition over the past 20 years. The industry has really changed, and I think it is continuing to change for the better as more information is learned and shared. I know that some of the things I write about in this book and some of the ideas I have will probably change, maybe even a week after I publish it. That is how fast the industry changes and how much more we learn about the body everyday.

My idea for this book is that you might relate to some of the things I have gone through physically, emotionally and professionally and maybe you can find some answers or save yourself from some of the mistakes I have made. Maybe you will be inspired to try some new things for yourself. Hopefully you will laugh a little and perhaps it will take you on a journey to learn more. I hope you enjoy!

Chapter 2 –ONE LOVE

Ahhhh One Love, my husband's least favorite term for this topic. This is one of my favorite topics, however, and is where we must start.

Your One Love is the reason you get out of bed in the morning, why you are who you are. It is what drives you, it is what motivates you to keep going and growing.

The idea of One Love has been a topic strung through my life and through the lives of the people I coach. A little more background on me: my husband and I have a son away at college. I can remember when he was shopping around for schools and taking his tests and telling me how the world works, because at 18 you pretty much know everything, right? I said something to him that my dad always said to me, "I know you better than you know yourself". Oh god I always hated when he said that to me, UGH!

Funnily enough, as I said it I really understood what my dad meant. It hit me at that moment when I was 40 years old. Ok so I am a slow learner, but I believe as we look inside sometimes, and question our abilities and our own strengths, especially when we are just about to head out on our own, we can't see who we are clearly. Sometimes it takes time to discover ourselves. Some do have a passion for something right out of the gate. Take my husband for example: he was an athlete, an impressive baseball and basketball player and he went right for health and fitness and coaching thru college and right from the beginning of his career. I, on the other hand, have done a lot of jobs and I have a lot of different interests. It took me awhile to discover that I love working with people, getting to know them and helping them discover their personal awesomeness.

Anyway, back to One Love; it's about passion, it keeps you inspired, it keeps you lit up and fired up! I have been a mom for many years, and that is how I identified myself, and it was definitely something I was passionate about for a long time. I loved laundry and making dinner and going to sporting and school events. I was really absorbed in it, even throughout my son's high school career. Then in a flash it was over.

It's the cruel joke of motherhood: you have this little helpless thing that you protect and take care of and then one day they scorn you and leave you! Ok maybe scorn is a little harsh, but they just up and leave, and you can no longer protect them or be involved in every little decision. The day my son went to college I said "My days as tour director are over". It's my time now. I am not going to say it's been easy because it hasn't. I miss being a full-time mom a lot (I will always be a mom, but I cannot be as nosey or bossy as I used to be, and I miss that). I have struggled with where I fit now. What is my One Love now that my first One Love left to live his own life?

I work with clients in the throes of motherhood, school meetings, driving to sports, making dinners and lunches, and just trying to find a minute for themselves. She plans a "date" with her husband, making time and making sure they keep time to themselves to stay acquainted. Making sure they don't drift too far away during these years with kids, so they aren't sitting in rocking chairs staring at each other! Moms and dads who are trying to keep it together day in and day out, and in a constant state of change. It's hard to believe in those moments sometimes that it is only a moment in time, and it will change before you know it. This is why keeping a sense of your own passion and your own self is so important.

Many times as parents, or even just as people, we wrestle with our own One Love. Like I said before, it's hard to see sometimes what we are best at and what we are passionate about, as we have children and parents and spouses all vying for our time and attention. Jobs change, kids grow up, parents grow older and pass on, and we are always changing whether we like it or not. This is another reason why it is SO IMPORTANT to find out what excites us and inspires us as we can ground ourselves in these things as everything changes.

Another client was talking to me about what it's like when the kids are grown up and gone. There is so much time to do whatever you want, like paint or golf or get blind drunk during the day. I know it sounds crazy, but more and more this is happening to women when they have spent their life caring for others and then they find themselves alone with all this time on their hands. This is another reason our One Love is so important! I have worked in gyms where old men would come in and just walk on the treadmill; no goals, no intention just walking the time away. Truly killing time.

Finding your passion is the most important to help keep you motivated to reach your goals and to keep you inspired to learn and grow for your entire life. Trust me, you do not want to be that person on the treadmill just killing time. I use One Love in the very first meeting with my coaching clients. I like to find out what their passion is, what is their dream? I can use this information to help motivate them to get healthy! You have to be healthy so you can do the things you love to do for a long, long time.

Sometimes it's hard to figure out what your dream is; we put so much into other people's dreams that we have lost sight of our own. I believe that everyone has a passion and a purpose. When trying to figure out what you love and what drives you, try to remember back to when they were young, before weddings and children, who were you then? What did you love to do in high school, what made you fly out of bed in the morning? These are questions I ask my son even now as he is well into his college career. It is a question you should constantly be asking yourself. Careers evolve (hopefully) and things change, we change. When you live your life with the intention to learn and grow every day, some things may get old and you may want to strive for something new. Your One Love may stay within the same genre, but how you deliver your message or go about your daily duties might change. There may be instances where you tire of one thing and jump into something entirely new. I would have never expected myself to write a book, but here I am doing something in the same field, but different!

Another way to approach finding your One Love is to think about your nightmare: what are you most afraid of? Sometimes exploring these fears can bring out the fire and the drive. When I have a client that does not know what their passion is and I ask this question, a lot of times these folks fear being alone. They have built their lives around others: their kids, their spouse, sometimes even their crappy job that they hate but are afraid to lose. I always tell these clients that they are never alone; you are never alone because you have yourself. These people need to be alone the most, to take some time out to listen to their own thoughts and stop junking up their minds with everybody else's drama.

It is scary to some, the thought of being alone with their thoughts. I have had a client break down crying after a yoga class because she never took time to cry after their dad passed away. We just block our emotions out and keep on trucking because that is what we **think** we are supposed to do, that we are weak when we cry and we have to be strong for our families. Sometimes others have to be strong for us. In order for us to be our best, we have to put ourselves first; I before we, always. You need to take care of yourself physically, emotionally, financially and mentally before you can be any good to your family, friends or otherwise. Sometimes you must be weak and vulnerable, otherwise you are just a shadow of who you are supposed be; no one is unbreakable. We are all human here. When that client broke down, I got to know her on another level, a human level, and we became good friends after that.

Journaling is another great way to connect with yourself and your dreams on a deeper level. Letting your mind go and wander, follow your stream of consciousness, write whatever comes to mind. Sometimes it's hilarious and sometimes it's very revealing. Stream of consciousness writing is something I do often and I journal every day, even if it is just a few lines on the paper. I love looking back and seeing who I was back then; sometimes I feel like I change on a weekly basis! My ideas and what I think about are odd or funny. They help clue me in to who I am now, and who I was. I create an awareness for me. In some instances, journaling is easier for people to do than meditation and I believe free writing or doodling is meditative. If you ask some of my Holistic Lifestyle participants, they will say one of their favorite activities I do with them is Mandala coloring. I break out the markers and the crayons and we have an old-fashioned coloring bee. We are creative beings living in a done-for-you world. We type on computers or watch TV and rarely ever get a chance to really get back to basics. Some people think The Kardashians are really reality. Yikes. Some would even say that is art, double yikes. We rarely even get the chance to take a breath and get to know ourselves.

It's part of the conspiracy if you ask me, but that is another chapter and maybe another book!

So what is my dream? I am a work in progress. I have worked for other people's dreams for a long time and I don't regret it one bit. I am definitely one of those people who didn't know exactly what I wanted to do when I was young, so going with the flow and taking the opportunities before me has helped me learn who I am. Writing also helps me explore my creativity and it sparks new ideas for new endeavors. I know I really enjoy helping people become better inside and out, and I love getting to know people on a deeper level.

So the message of this chapter is to dig deep, take a little time before your read on and think about who you are and what you want your life to be. What are your dreams? Write them down or draw them. Put them somewhere where you can see them at all times. Use your big dreams to guide you on your journey to excellent health! The most important thing is that, no matter where you are in life, you need to know yourself; you need that space just for you. Your One Love IS in there, so find it and use it. The force is strong within you!

CHAPTER 3 – WHAT YOU VALUE

When you establish your core values and belief systems they can help you define who you are and can give you direction and motivation to help you figure out your One Love. Values are the things that you think are important. They are present every day in the way that you conduct yourself and by the decisions that you make. Your values are reflected by how you look, who you hang out with, what you do for work and for fun. They are ever-present and some of your values probably change over time. What you valued at age 6 changed when you were 18, and from 18 to 30 et cetera.

Damon and I have a grown son in college. Throughout his young life and his high school life we attempted to instill our values in him while he was with us, hoping they would serve him well while he is out on his own. That's our job as parents, right? Its really hard to let go of being that person who told this other person how to live and what to do, to just listening to the choices and decisions that they are making and trying not to place too much judgment on them. Hey, it's their first attempt, we all made mistakes (and continue to in some cases). It's interesting to me to see how he thinks and how that relates to what we have tried to teach him as far as our values are concerned.

As a side note, it is funny for me to watch my husband get so frustrated with Nico when he doesn't comb his hair or portray a neat appearance. Looking sharp has always been a value of Damon's. Nico, being on his own this first year and not wearing his high school uniform all the time, and being in control of his own schedule, it appears that staying up late with friends and then sleeping until the last possible minute might be one of his values right now. He does not really schedule time to pick out his outfits or even comb his hair sometimes. Combing my hair and looking neat when I am in public is a value of mine, and I believe if Damon had hair it would be one of his. I do believe appearance will become more important to Nico as he adjusts more to his newly experienced environment friends and freedom. Independence won't be amazing once the novelty has worn off.

When Nico was living at home, crazy as it may sound to you, one of us always was always there in the morning to make him breakfast and say goodbye to him before he left for school. Even when he was in high school and plenty old enough to make his own breakfast; but if you have teenagers most of them just leave without eating breakfast. That would have been him. He is a smart kid and he gets As and Bs and there have definitely always been areas where he could improve his academics. I think we used to get more upset if he didn't eat breakfast than if he got a C. We value health, clearly, and we'd better, it's our business. I know that health is important to Nico; it is one of his values that he acquired from his time with us.

It's sad to say that, the more the parent values the grade or the college their child is getting into, is more the tendency to look away from the waistline of that child. So we create people who can achieve and get a job, but if health is not important and healthy habits are not important, the child becomes fatter and sicker and more depressed as they age. Great, you got a raise and DIABETES! AWESOME!

I need you reading this to understand that our value is not perfection or a size 0 or a 29 inch waistline. It's not about how you look; it's about your health. Period. You can tell yourself or your kids that they are beautiful no matter what and that is true, and you love them no matter what. You or they are beautiful at any size, but are you healthy? Are you making good choices for your health or are you eating ice cream every night and whining how your knees hurt? Personal responsibility is another core value of ours. One of my favorite quotes is from The Alchemist is "Be conscious of you choices and responsible for your action"... what a concept.

Now as Americans we value our lifestyle...our Rock and Roll Lifestyle. Money is the goal, money is the objective, money is what we value-money and stuff. I am sure that perspective changes if you are in a hospital bed or you can't move around to play with your kids, or when you get older and are too sick to travel to their wedding or other event. As my father would say, "We need to get our priorities in order". It's not a good idea to value health when it has already passed you by. It is important make the choices today so you can enjoy your tomorrow. Every day that you wake up you have the opportunity to choose health or sickness. You can choose to be a victim or you can take action to live the life you have always dreamed. Each of us has more power than we even can comprehend; instead of complaining about your health, do something to change the way you feel. In these days of Facebook posts and status updates I want to throw my computer out the window when someone goes on a public rant about how sick or helpless they are, trying to garner pity from their virtual friends. I want to comment and say "How is that working for ya?" Value your health, value your power, because when you change your values you can really make remarkable changes in your life.

Don't get me wrong; academics are important, achieving is important. It is not my goal to have my son living in my basement at 30 years old, and fortunately I am sure that's not what he wants either. In Nico's first year at college I told him that the tour director, being me, has completed her job. It is now time for him to take the steering wheel of his life and start to take responsibility and drive. I told him he was welcome to come back home if he could not manage to keep his grades at the level at which he needed to maintain his financial aid. One thing I knew is that once that child got a taste of independence and all the action that went with being at college, he would do what it took to stay there. I mean, really, what 19-year-old wants to live with two 40-somethings eating kale and going to bed by 10pm? This is his time! Another core value that we have tried to instill upon this kid is to get up, work it AND enjoy it, and also be independent. The only person you can count on to take responsibility for you is you.

I imagine you are reading this book because you are making a change in your life in some way. As you may have noticed, I coach by doing. I am not going to write about or suggest any of my clients do anything that I haven't tried as an option. I will write about my successes as well as my failures and let you know that I am not a perfect size 2, sometimes I don't even feel like working out, imagine that! Personal values of mine include honesty and integrity in my life and in my business. I try to be transparent emotionally too, as you will read in chapters to come. That is part of my commitment to being an honest and open coach. Some of the more personal things I have shared have gotten the most response from my clients and readers. Our experiences knit us together as well as our values. I find that your values will attract people of similar values into your life.

Take this into consideration, especially if you are looking for a romantic partner. Say you don't drink alcohol and you are interested in eating healthy and working out, you probably don't want to go looking for a potential partner at a bar where the main food is fried and the main activity or purpose there is to get drunk. Talk about looking for love in all the wrong places!

Values are so important to define for this reason. It really isn't as much about "the law of attraction" as it is really knowing what you stand for. Remember the old saying "You better stand for something or you'll fall for anything"? So many people get into relationships when they don't even know who they are. They fall in love or fall in convenience with whoever is there at the time because they don't want to be alone. You wake up 20 years later and say you are the health nut and you have figured out what excites you (One Love), and you are not afraid of it anymore, and your partner is that beer drinking biker that wouldn't set foot in a gym if there was a Harley sale. 20 years can be a hard web to get out of, not to mention all the time you lost just floating through life.

Let me tell you from experience coaching clients through situations like this, once you find out what you love and who you are and you start making changes in your life, sometimes it puts a cramp in your family life. The client starts losing weight and feeling happier while the spouse or family member stay the same. Those family members can get really bitter and mean. It is really hard for people to continue to make healthy changes in their life when the most important people in their lives are knocking them down. These people either quit making changes or they move on from the people that can't accept the new lifestyle changes. I have seen both scenarios play out. If you don't live out your own truth or your own dream, your life can be a life of feeling like a victim and never being fulfilled. Values are extremely important to establish in order to live a happy healthy and wicked awesome life.

Keep in mind, I am not saying your partner or your family has to be just like you. I am only saying that mutual respect for each other and each other's values is important in any relationship. Even your children, as they get out on their own, it is important to respect their choices and their point of view, even if it does include not shaving for weeks at a time. The sure way to drive your adult kids away is to offer unwanted advice, nag them and continually judge or critique their choices.

Fortunately values are ever changing, so personal hygiene will hopefully work its way back into my son's life. There is always hope, and until then I will bite my tongue.

You can establish values for your family, almost like your family code of excellence. I see painted decorative signs at Marshalls with lists of family values written on them and they are cute. They say things like "do your best" "work hard" and "respect others". Those are great ways to start a conversation with your little ones at home about what your belief systems are. We have core values at FFC too. I am not ashamed to say we got the idea from the Zappos company who prints their company values on their shipping boxes. Things like "Deliver a WOW experience" and "Bring your best every day". It's about being conscious of our objectives as a business and as a team. Why we are doing what we are doing, and how are we going to accomplish our goals as a team and as individuals. When we interview people, we make sure they jive with our values.

So what about being conscious of your objectives as a human and as a family unit? It's a worthwhile assignment for journaling and an excellent concept to explore at this point in the year. What do you value? What values do you hope to pass on to your kids or your community? Which ones have you already passed on? Answering these questions by yourself and with your partner or family will really tell you a lot about who you are. Doing so can also help you discover your desire in life, your One Love. Establishing values will set you on the path to attract more of what you want in life, and really get you on a path to whole-ness.

CHAPTER 4 - AIN'T NOTHIN' BUT A "G" THING

Have you ever felt addicted to a food? Like, say for instance Gummi Bears. Say you just love the chewiness, the flavor of that red dye #5 and there is something just so sweet about Gummi Bears, and you just keep eating them until you feel sick. Because Gummi Bears aren't really food, it's more like flavored plastic-y junk, but there is just something about them, right? Okay so it doesn't have to be Gummi Bears, I went through a phase last fall when I was addicted to Brussels sprouts. I ate them for lunch and dinner with nothing else, just straight up Brussels sprouts. I was addicted. I was making up recipes and making Damon eat them (he grew to like them, not so much for Nico, he wouldn't even try them). Eventually the phase wore off and I eat Brussels sprouts more responsibly now. That wasn't such a bad addiction. I have had worse...

I have been gluten free for a little over two years. If you are a coaching client of mine, or you have talked to me at any length over the past 2 years you know this. I am addicted to talking about it, rather annoyingly so. Now going gluten free is a journey, a journey through addiction, desire and temptation. First of all, the definition of gluten:

Gluten (from Latin *gluten)*, "glue" is a protein composite found in foods processed from wheat and related grain species, including barley and rye. It gives elasticity to dough, helping it rise and keep its shape, and often gives the final product a chewy texture

Everything good has gluten in it: pizza, pasta, beer, bread, pancakes, you see where I'm going here. Now what I have is a sensitivity to gluten. I haven't always had it; I used to eat all of those things with no problem. Let me clarify that I do not have celiac disease; that is more serious, that is a disease of malabsorption, where your body cannot absorb essential nutrients. What happens to me when I eat gluten was mostly digestive stress, I experienced leaky gut and all the glory that comes with that, bloating diarrhea (yay!), and I also get painful acne when I eat gluten.

Now I didn't realize how bad I felt until I really focused my efforts on not eating gluten. My skin cleared up and my bloated belly went away, which was a great feeling both physically and wardrobe wise. I could never understand why I always felt so heavy and bloated and tired, until I stopped eating gluten. It really took a good while for me to realize these benefits (and to realize how crappy I was feeling in comparison to how much better I felt off the "G"). It was so hard to say goodbye to eating like everyone else, especially on vacation. It's a choice that I make now, and believe me, I still slip up. I had a pumpkin whoopie pie that I could not resist while home this fall...pretty much worth the acne.

Now when I say I don't eat gluten, let me tell you what I do eat: not a lot of processed GF junk food. That is not what I am talking about AT ALL. Gluten free to me is eating organic grass-fed meats, organic fruit and veggies, bone broth of course, eggs, coconut milk, once in awhile a gluten free pizza at Pizza Fusion (the closest thing to the real thing that I have had) or some GF pasta, mostly quinoa, sometimes rice. I don't stock up on GF cookies and cake and crap.

A little more history on me, auto-immune disease runs in my family. In fact, my mother has rheumatoid arthritis and hypo-thyroidism and lives in constant fear of digestive distress - all of these are related to gluten intolerance, just google it! These immune disorders are highly hereditary; my great grandfather (my mom's side, obviously) had crippling arthritis. My grandmother also suffered from dementia later in her life, which can also be a byproduct of gluten intolerance (more on gluten's effect on your brain later). So anyway, my mom will not trade her addiction to gluten for health, she would rather take the medicine prescribed by the doctor that does not cure her, and it only keeps her relatively out of pain. I think one reason is because it's too hard to be different or she doesn't want to be viewed as picky. Also my mom's doctor should be telling her this stuff, but doctors don't make money from you eating a good diet. They make money from prescribing pharmaceuticals and having you come back to them for more every 5 minutes...don't get me started, because that's another whole book in my head. She has gotten a little better, but for her conditions, she really should be stricter in my humble opinion.

Ok, so what does this mean for you? I have read that about 40% of people carry the HLA-DQ2 and HLA-DQ8 genes, which make people susceptible to gluten sensitivity. There is a lot of hype and information out there about gluten sensitivity. In this chapter, I hope to shed some jargon-free light on this topic so that you can make the correct choice for you and your family. As you will read later on, this isn't just about acne and diarrhea, this is a matter of longevity and your health down the road. I would say that if there is auto-immune disease in your family, it might be worth a try for you to cut gluten out for a bit to see how you feel. Maybe you have no gall bladder or you have skin, liver, stomach or digestive issues, I would also say give it a go. It's not going to hurt you, and the choices to be made on a GF diet may help you with that tired feeling you get midday, and it may improve the numbers on the scale. I have had a client's nightmares stop when she went GF. You would be surprised at some of the ways our body is trying to communicate with us.

Also, I have recently read Dr. Perlmutter's book Grain Brain. This man is a board certified neurologist. He works with people with brain degeneration and diseases like Alzheimers and Parkinson's disease. He wrote his whole book about the relationship of gluten and brain degeneration, especially pertaining to insulin levels. We all know that insulin levels rise when we eat flour/wheat gluten containing products like, say, a bagel. Our body has to regulate the blood sugar and produce insulin to combat that over abundance of sugar or glucose that we just ate. It has been shown that normal to high blood sugar levels, even in people without diabetes, can cause brain degeneration, which is one more reason to check gluten off your healthy food list (Australian National University Study). The last time I saw my grandmother she didn't know who I was. She was in a nursing home and we were told she was saying things and doing things completely out of character for her. I don't want to forget my children or grandchildren. These kinds of diseases in my family are enough fuel for me to make that difficult change to gluten free.

So back to the addiction part: if you decide to try a GF plan, the first two weeks you probably will have cravings, and gluten stays in your body from anywhere between 2 weeks and 3-4 months! There is no halfway in with this plan, you are all GF or you are not. After two weeks, if you have symptoms like bloating or acne they may start to clear up, although it may take more time because you have been eating the other way for so long. If you are cheating a little bit, your symptoms will not clear up, it's that simple. It took a solid month of being all in for me to notice a difference digestively and with my skin, and now there is no turning back for me. I can't believe how I was living before, and I see my mom and know I don't want to live on medicine or take Imodium as precautionary action before any function.

As I said earlier, I still cheat once in a while when as Grammie Em would say "It's worth it", but in my normal everyday life, even on weekends, I am strictly gluten free. I generally can tolerate small cheats a couple times a year, but if I go overboard my body lets me know it with migraines and skin and digestive issues. Damon has also gone gluten free since listening to my monotony over the past two years and also because of the studies pointed out in Grain Brain. Being gluten free is part of our healthy holistic lifestyle.

We eat a lot more fat than we ever did before because of the research we have been reading about supporting healthy brain function over a lifetime. Of course I am talking healthy fat here, things like real grass-fed butter, avocados, olive oil the fat from grass-fed meats and especially coconut oil. Supplementing your diet with some coconut oil or MCT (medium chain triglycerides) is very supportive to brain health and function. In fact, your brain can quickly use the energy provided in MCT oil, because medium chain triglycerides go directly to your liver where that energy is immediately released into your bloodstream for consumption by your brain. Using MCT oil has been proven to restore and renew neuron and brain nerve damage even after damage has occurred! AMAZING stuff!

Don't be sad about giving up some of your favorite foods. There are so many websites with recipes so you can enjoy pancakes or pizza. I have a client who has made her kids go gluten free and she says that one of them is so much more chipper in the morning, she notices a real difference in their mood and energy! How cool! And the kids LOVE her recipe experiments!

Like I said, it's not necessary for everyone to go GF, but hopefully this chapter gave you some gluten free food for thought regarding this confusing topic. Omitting the gluten helped me, and if anyone else has symptoms like I did, maybe it won't take them 40 years to figure it out.

Also, if you are like me, and you are going to go GF, here is a recipe for BONE BROTH. I believe eating bone broth was essential to my gut healing progress.

BONE BROTH
You will need these items:
- A big pot or a big slow cooker.
- A fine metal strainer
- Glass ball jars or glass containers to store your broth
- Another big pot to strain it into
- A plastic and paper bag for trash

Ingredients:
- 4 lbs. of beef marrow or knuckle bones
- 2 parsnips
- 1 onion
- 5 cloves of garlic
- 3 carrots
- 3 stalks of celery
- 1 celery root
- 1 turnip
- Fresh rosemary, thyme, and oregano
- ¼ cup of apple cider vinegar
- Sea salt
- Water

Once you have gathered all your ingredients, you are ready to make some broth. Directions:
1. In a 400 degree oven, brown the bones on a cookie sheet or glass dish for about 45 minutes. Turn the bones over half-way through. Doing this adds more flavor and color.
2. While the bones are in the oven, cut up all of your vegetables into thick 1-2" pieces. They don't have to be pretty or perfect since you're not going to be keeping them in the broth. I will typically add the sea salt after it's cooked when I go to re-heat it.
3. Once the bones are done, place the bones in the pot and fill with water, leaving just the very tops of the bones exposed and bring to a boil for about 45 minutes.

4. After it has come to a boil, bring the heat down to low, and skim off any residue that's floated to the top.
5. After you've removed any scum at the surface, add your veggies and herbs, and fill with more water if necessary.
6. Let the brew simmer on super-low for about 4-6 hours stirring occasionally, and adding more water if needed.
7. After 4-6 hours of simmering, turn off your heat and let cool for a few minutes. Then, remove the bones from the liquid concoction and place into a plastic bag and place the plastic bag in a paper bag (trash).
8. Set your other big pot in a clean sink with your metal strainer sitting on top, and pour your liquid, straining all the veggies and herbs out.
9. Do this a couple of times, getting any bits and pieces left. Take what's been strained and put into the plastic bag in the paper bag.
10. Pour the liquid into glass jars or glass containers. This recipe usually makes about 3 glass Ball jars' worth of broth.
11. Let the broth sit in the fridge over night or for 24 hours. This will allow the tallow to form, which you will then remove before drinking. You can throw your tallow away, or like bacon fat, store in another glass jar to use for cooking.

Once cooled, the liquid will be congealed. When you re-heat your broth, use 6-8 ounces with a little bit of water. At this point you can add sea salt.

Bone broth contains minerals that can be absorbed by your body very easily. It also contains broken down pieces of cartilage and tendons, the stuff glucosamine and chondroitin are made of, so it's good for your joints and repairing our daily wear and tear on our bodies. It also contains valuable nutrients that help us heal and repair our gut walls, which in the end helps us with immunity and overall gut function.

CHAPTER 5 - IN THE LAND OF MILK AND HONEY

I have already mentioned in the introduction some of the habits and foods I ate growing up until the time I met my husband Damon in 1992. I drank whole milk and ate ice cream and pizza just like any other regular kid. So, as I said before, when I did meet my bodybuilder husband in college, he was shocked at how I ate! Especially the whole milk thing, that stuff sits on top of the cereal! Hey, it was the 90s and fat-free was the rage. At that time I began to put skim milk in my cereal, eat fat-free cheese and yogurt, all pasteurized and homogenized of course.

This low fat free/fat free thing is what we believed was healthy and good for keeping the fat off back then; fat makes you fat, right? Made sense at the time. We had a son in 1994 and loaded him up on skim milk and fat-free junk. Ugh sometimes I just wish I could go back and change what I fed that kid. Maybe he wouldn't be so addicted to Taco Bell. Maybe.

About the time I turned thirty I was starting to have my "doubts" about milk and its effect on me. I would just think about a latte and feel diarrhea coming on. I had to stop drinking milk. That is called listening to your inner voice, because if that voice says diarrhea, you listen. My body was never really great with ice cream so I had already started to avoid dairy.

So why is that? How did I become suddenly lactose intolerant? It has been proven that we lose some, or in some case ALL, of our ability to digest lactose past the age of four, the age when some cultures stop breast-feeding. Clearly I got along fine for 20-some years past 4 years old. What do they do to the milk now that might be different than 30 years ago?

Lets talk pasteurization. Pasteurization is the process that sets out to do two things: destroy disease-carrying germs and prevent the milk from going bad. They do this by heating the milk to a temperature of about 150 degrees for a half an hour. What the heck could be so bad in the milk that you have to cook it like that? Well, in our modern day and age of Bovine Growth Hormone to create bigger cows and higher milk consumption and the over milking of cows for much longer periods than they are meant to be milked for, with machinery that is painful to the cows but easier for the farmer, there is so much pus and blood that goes into that milk as it is coming out of the poor animal it is necessary to boil the heck out of it to get rid of those germs. Not to mention, when a cow gets an infection they pump it full of antibiotics, which also is transferred to the milk and then to us, making us more resistant to antibiotics when we get sick.

In the process of boiling out the bad stuff, you can imagine that the good stuff gets boiled out too. A lot of the valuable nutrients get destroyed, like vitamin C, vitamin B6, vitamin A and iron, iodine and folate as well. One of the reasons I probably became intolerant is because the lactase in milk is destroyed. The lactase is what helps you digest the lactose.

The FDA, The International Dairy Foods Association (IDFA) and the National Milk Producers Federation (NMPF) have now moved to allow companies to add aspartame or other non-nutritive sweeteners to milk and not label it on the packaging. Their reasoning is that it is a lower calorie option for the consumer. Yeah, lower calorie, higher health cost.

So how are we supposed to eat our organic, non-GMO Oreos you ask? Well there are a lot of options out there for people who cannot drink milk because they cannot tolerate it, or they don't want to drink milk because the whole pus and blood thing is just too disgusting. I use canned coconut milk now for any of my dairy needs; mostly for protein shakes but I have also made a killer whipped cream from canned coconut milk. I try to stay away from coconut milk or almond milk in a carton. The carton type has been known to contain carrageenan, which can add to inflammation of the gut. Not a good thing if you are trying to heal a leaky gut, also not a good thing if you don't have and don't want a leaky gut. I also make sure the canned coconut milk we buy is non-BPA, which is an endocrine disrupter, which can cause cancer. If you are a whiz in the kitchen you can actually make your own almond and coconut milk. There are recipes all over the Internet about that process.

Soy milk is something I try to avoid as well, actually soy in general. Soy products contain phyto-estrogens, which mimic the natural estrogen in our bodies. The leading cause of infertility, breast cancer and fibroids is an over-abundance of estrogen. It doesn't take a genius to understand that we clearly do not need extra estrogens from food. Soy suppresses the thyroid from getting the necessary iodine it needs to perform its duties. Thyroid issues are on the rise right now. People that have a hard time losing weight, fatigue, mood swings are all related to hypo active thyroid, but hey, medicine is big business, so let them eat soy right? Soy can also inhibit mineral absorption and our ability to digest proteins. This means more bad news for leaky gut sufferers.

You need to be vigilant in looking for soy in your food, sometimes listed as soy lecithin, it's in everything! I am sure back in the 80s Chips Ahoy and Cheese Itz did not include soy; they do now! Not that I am advocating these kinds of products for a healthy lifestyle, but even if you are buying treats for your kids you want to avoid soy. The reason you can find soy in everything now is because it's big business. The government subsidizes the production of soy, which was up until recently considered a waste product, a toxic waste product.

Soybeans are mostly all genetically modified (GMO) now too. Farmers purchase soybean seeds that are "Round Up Ready", which means the herbicide is already packed into the seed. Awesome. So now our food is modified to explode the stomachs of bugs, it probably won't hurt humans though. I am glad the government still gets its money at the expense of the people.

There are some people that argue genetically modified foods create a way to produce high volumes of food cheaper so we can feed the world. I am totally on board with feeding the world, but what are the consequences? Are we creating a generation that won't be able to reproduce? Is that the plan? Is a Brave New World closer than we think? Not to mention the degradation of our health and the health of those around the world. Is feeding people whatever is cheap, and who cares if it's healthy, the best idea? It will keep the pharmaceutical companies in business that is for sure.

I covered a lot in this chapter from dairy and pasteurization to soy and the evil that men/women do. I ranted a little bit on each of these and gave you a little information/opinion on each. Just like anything that

you read anywhere, you need to do your own research; there is a lot of information out there. I know how I feel eating these foods, and that is how I came to learn what I have shared here. You need to be aware of what you are putting in your body, every little thing. That is why I get so strict with my clients about eating whole foods; we all know what is contained in an organic strawberry. You know that if it is certified organic it has been farmed under acceptable standards and they haven't sprayed it with something that will give your future children a third (visible!) eye. The less you have to read labels and get around the tricks and lies of the regulators the better,
and most likely the healthier you and your family will be.

CHAPTER 6 – GET IMMUNE FROM THE INSIDE OUT

Since I have just spent a couple chapters talking about food sensitivities and leaky guts, lets dive a little further into the gut to further accentuate the importance of recognizing how different foods and situations can effect more than just your digestion. The state of your gut can have a major effect on your overall health as far as avoiding day-to-day nuisances like acne and migraines, to whether or not you get every cold coming down the pike or even something worse like cancer, or as I have already touched on Alzheimer's and other brain diseases.

So as you may or may not know, I live in sunny southwest Florida. We are so lucky to have about 360 days a year of sunshine. We get some major tropical heat in the summer and we get snowbirds in the winter. When these "birds" start flying down here for the winter they always tend to carry with them extra baggage from the plane, and by extra baggage I mean coughing, runny noses, diarrhea and puking, all the stuff fairy tales are made of, right? Now don't get me wrong; we love our snowbirds and we have missed them all summer long, but they know as we do that plane travel brings increased exposure to many germs that we would all like to avoid.

Of course you can probably tell by now, it is of utmost importance for me to stay healthy so I can work, play and live to my fullest potential! I want to not only be immune to coughs and flu, but I also want to build a strong system that can combat some more serious things like autoimmune diseases and cancer. We all want to improve the odds in our favor against the common cold and serious types of illnesses, right?

There are some signs and symptoms that you have digestive issues or a leaky gut and they are affecting your health and your immunity. Diarrhea, gas bloating, hormonal imbalances, allergies, autoimmune disease like thyroid disorders or rheumatoid arthritis, depression, and chronic fatigue can all be linked to a leaky gut.

So what exactly is leaky gut? It is exactly what it sounds like: undigested foods and particles permeate (leak through) the lining of your intestines because the lining has become weakened. The gut naturally lets very small particles through it so your body can absorb the nutrients provided by the foods we eat. In people who are sensitive, gluten can cause the gut cells to release zonulin, a protein that can break apart the intestinal wall lining and allow bigger particles to get through, particles that are too big to absorb. Other factors like infections, toxins, *stress* and age can also cause the intestinal lining to become compromised.

Once large particles are breaking through that lining, you have a leaky gut. When your gut is not functioning properly, things like toxins, microbes, undigested food particles, and more can escape from your intestines and travel throughout your body via your bloodstream. Your immune system sees these "particles" as enemies and begins to attack. Your immune system responding to these perceived enemies is what can cause the problems that I talked about previously.

As I have already discussed in the previous chapters, the main culprits for causing your intestines to become weakened are foods like gluten, dairy, excessive sugar or alcohol intake. Infections like candida overgrowth, intestinal parasites, and small intestine bacterial overgrowth (SIBO) can also cause problems in your gut. Toxic substances that we use everyday in the form of medications like Motrin, Advil, steroids, antibiotics, and acid-reducing drugs, and environmental toxins like mercury, pesticides and BPA from plastics can also contribute to the weakening of your intestines. Uncontrollable factors like stress and age also contribute to a leaky gut.

Leaky gut syndrome can cause the malabsorption of important micronutrients. The inflammatory process causes swelling and the presence of many poisonous chemicals, all of which can inhibit the absorption of vitamins and essential amino acids. A leaky gut does not absorb nutrients properly. Bloating, gas and cramps occur as do a long list of vitamin and mineral deficiencies. Eventually, systemic complaints like fatigue, headaches, memory loss, poor concentration or irritability develop. Not being able to absorb nutrients properly can also leave your body feeling like it needs to constantly fuel itself. What I am saying is that you are hungry very shortly after you have eaten a meal. Obviously, this can make you gain weight, and feel hungry and tired all the time.

So some very simple things that we do everyday can help us improve our immunity. Food choices are a big one, as you probably well know. Foods like coconut, kale and greens and supplements help keep your body strong and give your cells armor to protect against any "bad bugs" that might accidentally enter your system. Other healthy habits that promote immunity are meditation, proper rest and not beating the crap out of yourself at the gym (see the next chapter!). A lot of the choices we make every day either promote or inhibit our immune system's ability to fight off disease and keep us healthy.

One of my favorite memes says, "The main ingredient in hand sanitizer is paranoia." Our reliance on bacteria-killing CHEMICALS actually preys on our immune system rather than strengthening it. It's the same thing with gut health. Our reliance on antibiotics, or rather our obsession with antibiotics, actually promotes more serious diseases than it cures. We kill all of our own disease-fighting bacteria with antibiotics and hand sanitizer and wonder why we end up chronically sick or getting even sicker after "treating" our illness. Keeping healthy gut flora is essential to our health. Taking probiotics and eating fermented foods can help aid in keeping your gut healthy. Fermented foods are things like Kefir, sauerkraut, kombucha, pickles, coconut yogurt and miso.

As a side note, any kids born via cesarean section should definitely take probiotics, as they miss out on good flora that is transferred from moms to babies in the birth canal. Nursing your baby is a good solution for this because breast milk contains substances known as prebiotics that promote the growth of healthy bugs. They supply nutrients to the living bacteria and enhance their ability to survive and thrive in your child's gut. By shaping the content of an infant's gastrointestinal tract, breast milk also helps 'educate' the developing immune system.

Things that cause your gut to be out of balance in addition to taking antibiotics are taking other prescription medications, having been under anesthesia, consumption of too much sugar and acidic foods, and consumption of diet sodas or diet sugars like Splenda. Splenda is the trademarked name for sucralose, an artificial chlorinated sweetener that is formed when the hydroxyl groups in a sugar molecule are replaced with chlorine molecules. You know what chlorine does to your pool; imagine what it does to your gut!

Most of us (including most doctors) do not recognize or know that digestive problems wreak havoc in the entire body, leading to allergies, arthritis, autoimmune disease, rashes, acne, chronic fatigue, mood disorders, autism, dementia, cancer, and more.

Too many of the wrong bacteria, like parasites and yeasts, or not enough of the good ones, like Lactobacillus or Bifidobacteria, can seriously damage your health.
So if pharmaceutical drugs are in large part responsible for unhealthy gut flora, and having an out-of-balance gut can cause a whole array of different and very serious conditions that require even MORE drugs, who is benefitting by exacerbating this problem rather than solving it? Very rarely do I hear a client say their doctor suggested a probiotic to combat the negative side effects of their prescriptions. That would not be lucrative enough! Instead, with every illness and prescription, patients get mysteriously sicker and less healthy. I hear of more and more people with irritable bowel syndrome and food sensitivities. You wouldn't believe that people don't know that pooping every day, 2 times a day MINIMUM, is NORMAL!!! So many people are running around in a "diarrheal state of emergency" or with days of toxic poop hanging around inside of them. They can't poop one time a day, let alone two! And those state of emergency people don't even realize that poop should not be the consistency of yogurt, and it is not normal to have a 5-alarm fire coming out of your butt.

Here are some ideas to get (and keep) your gut on track:

- The very first thing I suggest is to do a detox or elimination diet. You need to get back to ground zero in order to figure out what is triggering your symptoms. This was a **life changing** event for me! Once I got clear of gluten, dairy, alcohol, caffeine, sugar, processed foods, legumes, eggs and meat, I could "test" back in each item to see how my body reacted. My skin cleared up, my digestion got better and I had a lot more energy once I got clear. My self-awareness has never been better as far as know what works for me and what doesn't. If I get a migraine headache now, I know EXACTLY what the heck I did to deserve it! Last time it was Norman Love birthday cake, so worth it though! Not all detoxes are as extreme as the one I did; you are probably thinking, "What the heck did she eat?" You can check out the back of this book for a link to my 21 Day Detox that is simple and defined. There are also awesome recipe ideas included so you can be sure you are not just drinking water for 21 days!

- Keep your diet organic and fresh and eat as much whole, non-processed food as possible. Lowering your intake of processed foods will keep your gut in check, and it will also make you take in fewer calories. Once you get "clean" your body should function more optimally. You will absorb more nutrients and your body will begin to feel satisfied. You should feel more satiated between meals, which means less snacks!

- Take probiotics every day either via foods, like kefir or kombucha or a supplement. A note on probiotic supplements: if you are just starting out on these, start with a 3 billion CFU (colony forming unit). This is your good bug army! You can work your way up from there. If you have EVER taken antibiotics, you need to replenish those good guys because antibiotics do not distinguish between good and bad. It is like the atom bomb of medicine. It just wipes everything out.

- Other supplements that I take to help my gut heal and stay healthy:
  - Omega 3 fatty acids to reduce cell inflammation
  - L-Glutamine to protect and restore the intestinal wall lining
  - Digestive enzymes just for a short time to help assist with digestion while your body is healing itself
  - Turmeric can help heal and seal your digestive tract. It also is helpful for lowering inflammation.

- Bone broth every day because it is just plain awesome for you! Also, it helps with strengthening your gut by improving digestion, and bone marrow helps the immune system by carrying oxygen to cells in the body.

- Washing your hands regularly with soap and water and forgoing the hand sanitizer. Hand sanitizer kills all the good stuff, too. Same idea as antibiotics...sound the alarm and get under the desk. It just wipes it ALL away.

- Eating my healthy green stuff. It's great for nutrition and hydration, and it just makes me feel like I am doing something good for my body. I don't want to delve too far into the POWER of POSITIVE THINKING, but believing you are healthy and taking action toward supporting a healthy self can do a lot towards keeping you from getting sick. You are what you say you are!

- Also, get enough rest and do not push too hard when you are tired. Sometimes a little less is better than WAY too much. This means you don't have to be the superhero every day at the gym or at work; listen to your body! If you need to go a little lighter or take a rest day do it, and get to bed on time. You need those 7-9 hours of recuperation each day!

Be aware that you have control over your life and your health. Once you go through the process of eliminating certain foods, toxins, and medications from your life you will be amazed. I walked around for a long time just believing that having emergency bathroom situations was just normal for me. Damon will tell you the story of my 40th birthday when we were sitting on the beach for my birthday getaway and he looked over at me while I was chugging Pepto-Bismol. Not my sexiest moment. I really believed this was my genetics! Hey, my mom has it, my sister deals with it, and we would just take Imodium and hope for the best. It's nice to not have to worry about that anymore!

I won't lie, giving up certain things like coffee and pasta sounds scary at first. I put off my first detox because I was downright afraid of coffee withdrawal. It was hard, but after a few days when the fog lifted and the withdrawal went away I felt lighter, more positive, and at the end of my 21 days, I had a new lease on my health. It really changed me in every way. I became empowered with my health! It may take you time or you may be in enough pain right now to decide to go for it. I encourage you to take the reins, you will be so glad you did!

CHAPTER 7 - MEDITATE, TRY NOT TO HATE

Just mention that word to a client and they look at you like you have three eyes! A lot of people have misconceptions about meditation, like: you have to shave your head, wear a robe and pass out flowers at the airport to do it correctly. They couldn't be more wrong.

I want to talk about why meditation is so important before I give you some SIMPLE tips on how to get some healthy meditation time into your day.

Probably the most obvious of reasons to meditate is that it lowers stress. Research shows that becoming more mindful is not only associated with feeling less frazzled, it's also linked to decreased levels of the stress hormone cortisol. Cortisol is a steroid hormone released in times of stress. Having an overload of cortisol can cause you to keep weight on and make you more susceptible to colds and illness. Practicing mindfulness can help you recover more easily from stress, like say your drive home from work, or a disagreement with your kids.

Meditation can also help you with digestive issues. We have all had that feeling of being nervous or anxious when you have an important interview or presentation. It is an emotion that we can feel deep down in our bellies, right? Some people get digestive distress when they are anxious or nervous, and some folks can even get stomach trouble when they feel sad or excited. Your stomach is so closely linked to your brain, your brain is responsible for your emotions and your stomach carries out the physical feeling. You have probably heard of having butterflies in your stomach? Even good feelings and happy emotions can be physically felt in the stomach. Taking a time out to just breathe (also good for digestion) can help to calm those nerves and set your belly right.

It is the same thing with stress eating. Many times we have feelings of sadness or anxiety that we don't know how to express for some reason. My clients often tell me instead of feeling these feelings they "stress eat" and swallow those feelings. We eat because we feel empty inside; we are trying to fill a hole. We are eating to try and feel satisfied. Many times I will tell clients to take a 5-minute emotional break when this occurs. If there is no physical reason to eat, like you just ate dinner but you still feel hungry, try meditating. Take some deep breaths.

To take these "belly feelings" a little bit further, lets talk about meditation for weight loss. So taking that break to decide if you are hungry for food or hungry for emotional expression is definitely advised before you reach for that snack. I have talked a lot about establishing awareness, and being aware and conscious of your feelings is paramount to losing weight and maintaining health. This is by no means a weight loss book, but part of being healthy is taking good care of our bodies; not perfection, a happy medium! Clients tend to believe that they must beat the crap out of themselves in the gym (See Chapter 8) in order to lose weight or stay healthy. What if beating the crap out of yourself is not at all what keeps you healthy? How about taking that time to "work in" and become aware, and not stuff our emotions down with a whole cake washed down with a bottle of wine while watching the Housewives of somewhere? Meditating can help you maintain an even keel, it can help calm anxiety, and the things that make you reach for the donuts and the alcohol. If you lose the donuts and alcohol, hey, you might just drop a few pounds and get a little healthier. You may even be more inspired (less hung over) to take a walk with your dog or play with your kids.

Sometimes adding a physically stressful workout to your life is more detrimental than helpful. Part of this awareness gig is knowing when to say when, as in the immortal words of Kenny Rogers, "you got to know when to hold 'em, know when to fold 'em, know when to walk away, know when to run". Know when to push yourself and know when you need to rest. I know sometimes I just don't want to work out, like if there are plyos on the program for the day and I am just being a baby. There are times when I just need an attitude adjustment and a workout usually does the trick. Sometimes, though, I am just not physically or emotionally up to par. Those days are good for extra meditation, a long walk in the sunshine or maybe just my stretching and mobility protocol. Knowing yourself is key. Don't be a wuss, but there is no need to be a hero either. The gym will still be there tomorrow.

Now I am not saying that meditating will immediately erase all your anxious or sad feelings without you having to express them. I count journaling as meditation too, especially if you are having trouble expressing yourself. In school we used to practice stream of consciousness writing, where you just sit and write everything that comes to your mind. It was used to help you get ideas and spark your creativity. I tell people to use it to get stuff out of their system. Sometimes we don't even really know what is bugging us. Some of the funniest stuff I have ever written is stream of consciousness. I have a client who had a hard time meditating, 3 kids 3 dogs, a fish a hamster, a husband, anyway, you get my drift. The easiest way for her to focus and meditate was to hide away in her closet and just write. She gets some of her best ideas in that time. It's a great way to discover your One Love too. I would say that a lot of times, stress is created from not having a creative outlet or a passion. We get so caught up in the day-to-day, we lose ourselves, and that day-to-day grind can make us anxious and beg the question "What is it all for"? Meditation and journaling can help us remember who we are, and set us in the right direction for happiness!

The coolest thing about practicing meditation regularly is that you can feel the benefits of it throughout the day, even when you are not actively meditating. I have really been making meditation a habit in my daily life and it has gotten so I really look forward to it. I practice for a half an hour every day. Now when my half hour is up my body naturally snaps out of the meditative state.

You have your own, unique brain wave frequencies: Beta, Alpha, Theta and Delta. Beta is your wide-awake mind, Alpha is your relaxed mind, Theta is your meditative mind and Delta is your sleep state. You can jump between all of these states during meditation or while attempting to meditate. The coolest state to reach in my opinion is Theta. Theta is that place between being awake and being asleep. It's a place where it feels like you are awake dreaming. It is the ideal state for meditating, because it is the ideal state for learning and memory, increased creativity and stress reduction. There is a great book simply called Theta by Bryan Jackson that has helpful exercises to get you in to that Theta state.

Sometimes I fall into Delta state during meditation, I always feel like I must have needed that nap! Some folks get worried that they will fall asleep while trying to meditate. Sleep is ok as long as it doesn't last 3 hours! That might mess up your regular sleeping pattern. That's why setting a timer is helpful. You allot for a certain amount of time and not get too caught up in the restfulness! If you are finding that you immediately fall asleep, take some time to think about why that is happening. Are you not getting enough rest at night? Maybe you need to get into your bedtime routine sooner. Are you feeling too much stress during the day? Maybe it is time for you to take a day off or schedule that vacation. Are you depressed and just want to tune out of your life altogether? Maybe you need a change or a new hobby, find something you love to do or schedule something fun to look forward to, or maybe you need to find someone to talk to.

Other great things meditation can help with:

- It can help to lower your health care costs
- It increases your immunity
- It can increase fertility
- It helps you sleep better
- It can help with depression

Hey what's not to like, right?

I know this all probably still sounds "woo woo" to you, but its really more simple than you might think. You can start with a goal of just 5 minutes a day. Set your phone timer and go sit outside in the sun, close your eyes and just listen to the birds. Usually it is best done when the lawn mower guy isn't out there tearing it up, so pick a quiet time of day. I usually meditate in the early afternoon after I have lunch. That time gives me a chance to let go of the morning and digest a little bit before jumping into my afternoon plans. I will put on some calm meditation Pandora Radio and just close my eyes and focus on my breathing.

Start with nice deep belly breaths, where you allow the air to fill up your belly before it rises to your chest. Belly breathing is so helpful because it takes us out of our forward posture, chest breathing, stressed out state and our body naturally relaxes when we practice belly breathing. Focusing on your breathing can help to clear your mind of your grocery list or whatever is floating around in there on any given day. It is ok if you do find your mind wandering to work or dinner or whatever, just come back to the breath.

Lying down with your back flat on the floor and your head just propped with a towel and your knees raised up on a pillow can help you relax and keep good posture. Sitting up is good too, but I like to recline, it's more relaxing for me. I am not trying to be Buddha or anything!

Another great tool Damon and I use for meditation is the Holosync series of mediation recordings. Holosync is soothing music, chimes and rain mostly that help to balance your brain. This method was what really got us to start practicing meditation regularly. The best thing about it is there is no clear your mind junk in here, its just click on your iPod (Holosync is most effective by listening with headphones) close your eyes and listen. Easy peasy. The other cool thing about it is it's a half an hour program, no worries about falling asleep for three hours; when the music clicks off, you click back on and feel pretty darn refreshed!

As a mostly hilarious side note, when I was a kid my dad bought these audio tapes for mediating and one was "Increase your Psychic Ability". I was obsessed with this tape. It was a guided meditation following a little squirrel through nature. I listened to it religiously for a while but never really felt any more psychic. To this day I wonder what squirrels have to do with being psychic or acquiring psychic ability.

Like I said before, start with small increments of time and work your way up. Make time for it in your schedule every day; it should be as important to your self-care plan as brushing your teeth! I promise, if you dedicate yourself to a regular practice you will be feeling the benefits in no time!

CHAPTER 8 – WORK OUT SMARTER

As you know, I am a personal trainer by trade and I co-own a small personal training gym. Helping people get and stay in shape has been my life's work for over 15 years. I have seen many trends come and go, thank god the thong on the outside of your pants has gone, like who thought of that one? Yikes! A trend that I see more and more of lately is using workouts as penance. For some crazy reason people think more is better, and crawling on the floor bleeding, sweating, panting, **puking** is what it takes. People think "Oh god I had a piece of cheesecake or a keg of beer this weekend, let me just go beat it out of myself at the gym this week" or "OMG the scale is up 1.2lbs, I better go lift, run, play tennis, swim walk, play twister and hate myself (all in one day may I add) until that pound comes off!" I have had new clients say to me "You aren't going to scream at me like Jillian does, are you?" That makes me nuts! The extreme behavior shown on reality TV and social media frightens people and keeps them from getting started on a road to better health through exercise. I once saw a program where the trainer made the new client puke and she kept telling the poor lady, "Oh that's just the toxins leaving your body." Now that is an advertisement for starting a fitness program if I have ever seen one, no wonder only about 25% of Americans work out regularly.

Don't even get me started on the new trend of competitive exercising. If you are into it, good for you, but I think most would agree, these kinds of lifts are not ideal for beginners (ask all the chiropractors, physical therapists and orthopedists getting rich off of Crossfit injuries these days). Did you know that the winners of the Crossfit Games actually have a strength-training program that they do in order to be good at Crossfit? Like training for a sport, they hire a trainer to create a program for them so they can be awesome at their "sport". Don't get your panties in a WOD –(Workout of the Day, I had to say that), I am not knocking Crossfit; if that is what you are into, awesome! All I am saying is it can be intimidating and maybe not the best place for people to begin their fitness journey, and if there is a puke bucket in the corner of the gym, maybe you should think twice about signing up.

Not to say you shouldn't work hard in the gym, but you should never feel like a steamroller has hit you. When you start a new program, some soreness should be expected, but you should still be able to go to work and lift your arms and sit on the toilet.

Lets talk fitness myths. I have clients that to this day, no matter how much we try to educate them, believe that cardio is the key to fat loss. Now I would say that Damon and I are in pretty good shape for our age. We NEVER do any sustained cardio, EVER! You will not catch me on a Stairmaster, elliptical, stationary bike for hours at a time; I have a life to lead! I have been in gyms where years will pass and the same person is on the same piece of equipment forever and they look THE SAME! You never see these folks pick up a free weight; they just plug along on the treadmill at 2.2 miles per hour or sweat their arse off on the elliptical, like they are training to be the most awesome ellipticalist ever and either their bodies never change or they get fatter and older looking. YIKES. People think that you have to spend hours at the gym on a road to nowhere, and this perceived investment of hours and hours of your life also keeps people from getting started. That goes for triathletes and marathoners too: they run and run and pound and pound their bodies, and if they don't practice strength training, they age themselves and hurt themselves in the end.

Some people, women and men alike, are afraid to lift weights. They think that if they lift anything more than 3lbs they will get "bulky" like those super tan fitness competitors in tiny bikinis that flex on stage. All I have to say to that is "if only". If you think it is that easy to get that fit, you need to go follow a fitness competitor around for a day. Eat what they eat, do what they do. There is SO much time, energy, self control, and discipline that goes into fitness competing, most of us could only keep that kind of regime together for maybe an hour. If it was that easy, more people would do it. I love when people say "I don't want big arms or big legs", then I say stop eating potato chips! Lifting weights will not make us big, but it will make us strong and resilient, and we'll have lower body fat as a side bonus!

Also, you cannot spot reduce, thank you Suzanne Somers. The thigh master and all those other infomercials are about marketing! How do you think she affords those bio-identical hormones? Fat comes off where it wants to and in time. There is no 4 minutes to a 24 inch waist and washboard abs. It takes dedication and commitment. There is no magic pill that won't give you some crazy side effects like anal leakage or eyeball rashes. There is no substitute for hard work, and it doesn't have to be hard; in fact I believe it should be fun! I resolve to bring the fun back to fitness!

Lets talk specifically about fat loss right now. There is a proper order for achieving and maintaining fat loss. The first thing to focus on is not even found in the gym, it's found in your kitchen. Eating good quality, not from a package, foods. Eating clean is our motto. The less you eat from a bag or a box the better. Focus on fresh organic veggies and grass-fed organic meats, and healthy fats like coconut and avocado. I promise, the more of these types of foods you eat, and the more you avoid sugar and processed foods, the more satiated your body will be. You will feel more energized and less hungry throughout the day. There is no magic diet, and if someone tells you there is they are trying to sell you something.

The next tier of the pyramid is to strength train! Like I said before, this doesn't mean picking up those dusty old 3lb neoprenes in your basement or any old random combination of exercises. The best results come from a structured and periodized program. The best programming that we have found for fat loss and for overall health is a combination of upper and lower body exercise in your program 2-3 times per week, along with some interval training which I will discuss as the next tier. These programs should change exercise selection and sets/rep range every 4-5 weeks (not every day!). These programs give your neuromuscular system a chance to get used to the exercises and also give you a chance to get stronger and progress. My clients love to see that their weights have increased in the 4-5 week period that they have been training. It's a great feeling of power and it makes you appreciate your body for all that it is capable of!

The more muscle you have, the more energy you expend just moving around during your day. Lifting weights can even afford you a few cheats through the week. You can enjoy a piece of cheesecake or a beer once in awhile. Your muscles will burn those extra calories off for you, no need to beat yourself up over it!

Being strong is so crucial to staying healthy physically and mentally. I know that when I am having a down day, just getting to the gym and seeing friendly faces and then focusing on my workout can help adjust my attitude in no time. Having a healthy and strong body makes me feel more confident and happy!

There are so many more benefits to strength training, more than just keeping the fat off. Another visual effect of strength training is postural improvement. Without strong muscles helping us fight gravity every day of our lives, our bodies tend to compress or shrink. We also can develop painful habits like a forward head and rotated shoulders. Staying strong and in alignment can help us stay tall and pain-free.

Strength training can also help us maintain our hormone balance. As we age, our natural production of hormones starts to decline. Growth hormone (our youth hormone) starts to diminish after age 26; strength training can help to boost those levels, and some goes for testosterone. On the other hand, strength training can "burn off" excess cortisol (stress hormone). Maintaining healthy body fat levels contribute to a better overall hormone balance, especially for females.

Other benefits of strength training include:
- It increases bone density
- It gives you better balance and body awareness
- It lowers your risk of diabetes and some cancers, including breast cancer
- It can reduce PMS symptoms
- It lowers cholesterol levels as well as blood pressure

The next piece of the puzzle is interval or metabolic training. As I said before, Damon and I don't do any long sustained cardio session, we focus on short burst training, interval training. So that means sprinting say for 30 seconds and then walking for 30 seconds, or we'll put clients on the dreaded airdyne bike for 30/30 – five times, and that is their interval training at the end of a strength program. Our boot camp or HIIT (High Intensity Interval Training) classes are made up of exercise stations that we rotate through for set periods of time and rounds. These classes last for a half an hour or so and you feel worked out at the end! No need to spend hours and hours at the gym. And if you are adding this style of interval training to your strength training, all that muscle helps to keep your fires burning all through the day. I have had clients say they were still sweating after lunch time from this type of workout!

The last and least effective type of exercise for fat loss is long sustained cardio, which is not to say don't do it, just know if you do it its not the most effective way to burn calories. These are activities like running, biking long distance, or elliptical like I mentioned before. I have some clients that just love to run, you know those "runner's high" types, and that is great, these people strength train a couple times a week and they just run because they love it. Without strength training, these types of activities just promote overuse injury, stress and early aging.

With all that I just said about exercise, it is important to keep in mind the previous chapter that I wrote on meditation, or working in. Regeneration and recovery are so vital for good health, as important as working out if not more so in our stressful world. We factor in a day of recovery each week where we will just walk or relax. Working in a gentle yoga class or Tai Chi can help to offset your tough week of workouts and get your body and brain relaxed and stretched out. It is so important to know when to take a break. We also suggest a week off every 12 weeks. It is important to give the body a rest, and a lot of times a week off can be plateau buster too! If you are feeling extra sore or extra tired, take a day off. Remember, working out is about self love and self care, not abuse.

My best advice on getting started is to hire a good trainer. They can put together a program for you to get you started and keep you motivated. Like I said before, make sure you are working the same 1 to 2 programs for 4-5 weeks. If they are throwing something different at you every time, it will not give your body a chance to improve. If hiring a trainer is too much of an investment for you, you can sometimes find programs online; Damon and I have put together a 42 Day Transformation
Program that comes complete with strength and metabolic workouts and videos you can follow along with. Rest days are even factored in

as well as meditation tips. There is actually so much more included, like nutrition advice and recipes as well as a detox. You can find more info on purchasing this program at the back of the book in the references section.

CHAPTER 9 – BEAUTY AND THE BEASTS

So trying to live a more holistic and healthy lifestyle does not mean you have to grow a full beard and run around smelling like a gorilla. There are so many great, natural products out there to help you stay looking good, smelling good and staying healthy while you do it!

I am finally getting the hang of this non-chemical deodorant and all natural beauty products thing. I decided to stop using my regular DEGREE deodorant. It did happen to be the week after I returned from Costa Rica and developed Dengue Fever. Yes, fever, which means I was sweating like a horse for a little over a week. Granted, I was in bed for about a week and a half trying to recover, but during the moments where I rallied, I was showering and only using all natural, paraben-free deodorant.

Why I chose that moment in time I still don't know. Poor Damon. Not only was I constantly tossing and turning and going between ice packs and heating pads and TRYING to stay hydrated, I did not smell like a rose. Needless to say, when you are making a change, you have to do it when the time is right for you, and boy did I put those deodorants to the test!

So why did I do it? You may or may not know that deodorants contain a lot of suspect chemicals, chemicals that can disrupt your hormone function. There are no known studies where the use of deodorants with aluminum, parabens, and triclosan directly cause cancer. It has been shown that exposure to some of these products can cause elevated estrogen levels. Aluminum particularly has been shown to mimic estrogen; elevated estrogen levels have been tied to higher risk of breast cancer. Aluminum, which is also found in most deodorants, can also affect your nervous system.

Not to mention, have you ever just shaved and maybe cut yourself a little and then you put on deodorant and it feels like 1 million fire ants burning up your skin? That just cannot be good for you!

Now that the fevers are over, I am having some success with the all-natural deodorant. I do use two different kinds daily and I do re-apply. The two I have been using are the aluminum free Thai Crystal (be careful, some crystal deodorants still contain aluminum!) and EO Organic lavender scented deodorant spray. They work great for normal, everyday activity. During a workout this week I was starting to offend myself, but I did take a poll of those working out with me and no one else noticed. I have also used coconut oil for deodorant and I have read that apple cider vinegar also can be used, that is if you don't mind running around smelling like a salad. Keep in mind with all natural style deodorants that they will stop the smell but not necessarily the perspiration, as in caution you might get wet. Interestingly, none of the contents of sweat stink; it's the bacteria on your skin's surface that interacts with sweat produced by the apocrine sweat glands to produce the smell. If you are stinky, it can be a sign that you need to drink more water (or eat less garlic).

I have been using organic body creams for a while now. I use organic body cream and I sometimes use coconut oil. I don't use coconut oil all the time because you can overload and become allergic to it...overexposure, especially if you are ingesting other coconut products. On my face I use jojoba oil, which I know sounds crazy but my organic facial person recommended it and I found I really like it. It's not greasy at all, like you would expect an oil to be. She does not recommend coconut oil on your face because it can cause your skin to break out in little whitehead zits. The best thing you can do for your skin is drink a lot of water and clean up your eating habits. You cannot put anything topically on your skin that will help with acne problems. Take it from me; I bought every Proactiv item under the sun and they never worked for me the long term. Don't believe the lie that birth control pills will help your skin. If your hormones are causing you skin problems, there are other things to explore to CURE your problems (and internal inflammation), not just put a Band-Aid on it!

I would like to take a moment to step up on the soap-box with regard to birth control pills. Doctors put girls on birth control pills when they are 16 for reasons other than avoiding pregnancy, things like acne or heavy, crampy periods. Girls stay on the pill for 15 years, and then want to get pregnant, and find that they can't. They have just messed with their natural cycle for 15 years, I don't know how one could expect that all would be fine after that length of time. Then you have to see another doc for expensive IVF or other hormone treatments. I also believe that they set you up for daily pill taking for a reason...because all this messing with hormones can affect things like your thyroid, PCOS problems; they get you in young and keep you in their clutches!!! My advice: find out the cause of the problem. Tell your daughters if they want to have sex, protect themselves with condoms! If they want to get rid of acne, stop eating processed crap out of boxes and bags and quit drinking soda and monster drinks. Find the root of the problem! Don't just automatically medicate. Quick fixes are never the answer; just talk to the woman who cannot get pregnant. Going through those treatments is emotionally painful, the worst kind of pain. Ok, stepping down.

I do not use regular toothpaste either. I use Tom's of Maine and a little baking soda. I also oil pull, which means, taking a teaspoon or so of coconut oil and swishing it through your teeth for 20 minutes or so. It is a very weird and time consuming thing, but I do find I get results from it. Damon said my teeth were looking whiter and I also feel like my gums feel better, especially if I have a sore spot from food getting caught between my teeth.

Making the toothpaste change is a big one, though, when it comes to overexposure to fluoride. Fluoride is actually banned in China, Japan and the Netherlands, and nearly all of the European water supply is fluoride free. High levels of fluoride in the body have been shown to cause Alzheimer's disease, lower IQ, early puberty, and thyroid dysfunction; it damages bones and the Nazis used it to cause docility in prisoners. Not only is fluoride in toothpaste, it's in the water supply and can be found in processed foods! Fluoride toothpaste was one of the first items I removed from my repertoire.

In my old age I am trying to wash my hair less often, and this is a hard road as I have very fine, very "tends to be oily/greasy" hair. The less often you wash your hair the less frequently your body has to produce more oil to keep your hair healthy. I have even read that having too dry hair (from washing too much) can lead to baldness; I bet Damon wishes he had had known THAT in the eighties. Now there are some hard-core holistic gurus that use baking soda and apple cider vinegar rinses on their hair and that is all. I really feel I may be little too conventional for that, although I may soon try replacing one shampoo a week with this method. The recipe is 1-2 tablespoons of baking soda in warm water in a bottle, mix it up and put it in the shower. You dump this on your head when you take a shower, massage it in (it won't foam up on you so beware of that) and thoroughly rinse it out or you could have volcano lava on your head once you spray on the ACV. Then, add a tablespoon of apple cider vinegar to a cup of water in a spray bottle. Spray this on your hair and rinse it out.

Castile shampoo can be another method to try if you don't feel like cooking up the baking soda/vinegar method. You can also find some other acceptable all natural brands of shampoo out there. I am still looking for something that works well for me. Fortunately, I have my hair long now and ponytails work if the shampoo doesn't. Additives that I try to avoid are any ingredients like ammonium laureth sulfate and glycol. Just like in deodorant, these are cancer-causing agents that should be avoided. Also polysorbates, which can disrupt the skin's natural ph, and dimethicones, which are found in conditioners and make it more difficult for the skin on your head to breathe.

I have cut WAY down on other products like mousse and hairspray, since I am washing my hair less, the more junk I put in it, the more I feel the need to wash it.

Its pretty much the same with make-up: stay away from products with parabens and "eth" ending ingredients. Look for products that are made from organic food grade, plant-based materials.

Let's talk sunscreen too: titanium oxide or zinc oxide is your safest bet to protect your skin if you are going to be in the sun for a longer period of time. Neither of these products penetrate your skin's surface. About 15 minutes of unprotected sun time is ok and considered good for you, especially if you are fair-skinned; you can go a little longer the darker your complexion. You may think tan skin looks good but actually, it is a sign of damaged skin. Most people absorb plenty of vitamin D in 15 minutes of sun time. Absorbing some sunshine into your skin can help us avoid diseases like cancer, diabetes, heart disease and depression. When Vitamin D levels are low, the hormone that controls appetite slows down, making us feel hungrier than we actually are.

It is not always easy to avoid chemicals in our beauty products or even our surroundings. Making informed choices and even just cutting down on some of the things you use daily can help you to live a healthier lifestyle. Minimize the risk, as they say in the insurance industry! Like everything else I have talked about so far it's about trial and error, find out what works for you.

Some of these choices that we make surrounding our beauty we have to realize are being sold to us by magazines, TV and the internet. One of the healthiest things you can do for yourself right now is to look in the mirror and accept yourself, for all that is past and present and for what is to come. Love those laugh lines and stretch marks, they tell the story of your journey! Those ideal bodies in the magazines are so airbrushed and unreal. You are real, and you are beautiful, just the way you are!

CHAPTER 10 – COME ON GET HAPPY

I am going to end this book with what really is the beginning of your journey, mostly because this concept is what will get you started on the road to a more holistic lifestyle, and it will sustain you on the right path for years to come. This concept sounds like a simple one, but it does require some soul searching for a lot of us, me included.

First, let's talk about what it means to live a holistic lifestyle. It should really be called a "wholistic lifestyle", as it is not solely about nutrition or exercise, although those things are very important. It really is about encompassing everything in your life, and for me it's the true path to happiness. When you feel happy, you are more likely to want to take care of yourself and maintain your health so you can maintain your happiness and keep doing what you love (One Love!). Although healthy eating and regular exercise is a great place to start, they will only take you so far on that path.

When my son was deciding on his college major I kept asking him, What is it that you could get so engrossed in that you forget to eat and sleep? And I don't mean a girl, like we all know that kind of love only lasts so long! What are you so passionate about that time just slips away? Anything can be made into a career. Don't focus on the money, focus on the feeling and the excitement, that kind of passion. I know that money cannot buy you happiness; I see it all the time. Trust me, living simply and loving what you do rather than cursing your alarm every morning is way better. Its like Tony Robbins says, "Live with passion."

As you may know, things change over the course of a lifetime. Priorities change, situations change, and what you love today may change many times over a lifetime. That's why it is important to be open to trying new things and meeting new people. Change is one of the only constants in life, and it's important to be willing to embrace change and go with it! My life is changing as I write this; my kid is grown up and getting ready to start taking care of himself without our help, and that is a big change for me. Letting go of that motherly control, learning how to butt out, is a big adjustment for me. Some days it's easier than others, but I know over time it will be normal, and my focus will shift from him to something else.

One of the other constants in your life is you; you will always have you. You need to take care of you first, that is why I am so passionate about good health. As long as I take care of me I can always deal with anything or anyone that comes my way. One concept that is hard for some people to grasp is "I" before "We". You must always take care of yourself before you can take care of anyone else. I think people have lost sight of the fact that we have control over our health and our lives. We become overly dependent on others to tell us what is good for us, when if we just got quiet and cleaned up our diet and made things simpler, we innately know what is good for us. The small choices we make every day affect every part of our health and ultimately our happiness.

Health-wise, in order to be happy there are a few very important steps: my final recommendations I would like to reiterate as I bring this book to a close.

Lets talk a little about sleep. First of all, it is very hard to maintain happiness when you are overtired. Anyone who has ever been around an overtired toddler knows this. As adults, we may not cry and throw our sippy cups, but we definitely are not the best we can be on too little sleep. I suggest 7-8 hours of sleep every night. If that's not possible, a little catnap in the daytime can help. It is important to maintain your circadian rhythm (sleep rhythm) to maintain healthy hormone and stress levels. The first four hours of your sleep period focuses on physical repair, healing and healthifying your body. In the second half of the sleep cycle, the focus is psychological repair, resting those brain cells that will help you make good decisions and solve problems all through the day. You can see why this sleep cycle has such a profound effect on your happiness quotient. If you are not clear-headed and your body feels sore, it's a lot harder to be happy.

Now we get to the more obvious stuff: You need to fuel the body for happiness. I always recommend my clients eat organic produce and grass-fed organic meats. I also suggest that they eat very minimally out of boxes, bags and packaging of any sort. I advise them to stay away from gluten, as for most people these days there is some sort of sensitivity, not to mention these kinds of foods just tend to be calorie-laden and slow us down. It is also good to avoid genetically modified ingredients such as corn and soy.

I always advise my clients to drink half their body weight in ounces of clean, pure water. I know when I am dehydrated I feel very slow and foggy and not really that happy. It is SO important to be aware of how certain foods, choices and habits affect you on a day-to-day basis. Really being accountable for your choices when it comes to food can make a huge difference in how you feel and ultimately how happy you are.

Pay attention to your poop. You will know how different foods, or even dehydration, can affect you if you check out the toilet bowl from time to time and see if everything is "altogether" healthy, or if you may need to change things up or take things out of your diet. Pooping should not be difficult and it should not be urgent. If either of these problems are happening, your body is sending you a message that you should stop and listen to. If your belly doesn't feel right, it's really hard to be healthy and do the things you want to do.

Movement is also an important part of the happiness game. We were just talking this morning during our Team Training about how you can walk into the gym feeling not so great, but you always walk out feeling better. For me particularly, it's a great attitude adjuster. Whether I am feeling angry or sad or just not quite myself, a good workout with some friends at the gym always puts things in perspective and returns the smile to my face. Your body releases those feel good hormones that send a message to your brain to snap out of the funk! Even just getting a leisurely walk in during the day can just make that much of a difference to change your perspective and happy you up!

Lastly, we need to connect with others and nature more often. Somewhere along the way, Facebook and cell phones have taken the place of real connections, and that has taken away some of our happy. We also get so engrossed looking down at our phones that we actually miss the beauty that is right in front of us. I have been to concerts where people are so busy recording the performance that they are missing the live event that they paid to see. If I wanted to watch a recording of the performance I could have stayed home! Look up people! I recently read a quote that said, "True love is when they put the phone down for you." Because of this technology, we have gotten so we work no matter where we are, all the time. If you have ever seen the movie "The Shining" you know that "All work and no play" is very dangerous! I am just as guilty as the next person of being too plugged in. I have made a habit of leaving my phone at home if I am going on a "date" with Damon, and I also try to only answer emails in the morning and at night, twice a day. We actually always talk about going off the grid. Studies show it takes 4 days to really get your head disconnected from technology. Besides, I have never heard anyone say "I had such a great time scrolling through Facebook last night". Computer and phone time is not living; it may be necessary but it is not what is going to make your life memorable. In the end, memories are all we really have.

Getting out and meeting people is tough in this day and age. Some of the best friends I have I found at the gym. I find these people are positive and on a similar path, looking to get better everyday. One of the things that takes away from our happiness is if we have negative or destructive people in our lives. It's hard to grow and make positive changes if someone is always raining on your parade or trying to get you to "eat that cheesecake" or "drink that beer" when you are trying hard to make changes in your life. Sometimes people need to be left behind, and that can be hard to do, but sometimes it just happens naturally. As you make changes and your priorities change, your path changes and naturally leads you away from things and people you just don't "jive" with anymore. The more positive and healthy you are, the more attractive you will be to other positive, healthy people. Like attracts like!

Once you get happy and you make more actual people connections you can really share the happiness, which will make more people happy. Just a random smile at Starbucks can make someone's day. You just never know how you can affect someone. Can you imagine if we were all happy and taking responsibility for our health and happiness and sharing our talents and happiness?

I also advise you to go outside, turn off the Netflix and connect with the earth. Take off your shoes and walk in the grass, take a walk on the beach or take a hike. Getting out and just breathing in the fresh air and taking in some beautiful scenery is good for the soul. Some of the best memories I have are from camping trips or hiking with friends. I have also met some great people and learned a lot about the world and myself by going on outdoorsy adventures. Connecting with nature brings us back to what is real, and where we come from as humans. It is so easy to forget that as we stare into our computer screen every day. There is so much out there to enjoy and explore.

I hope this was a helpful book. I really believe things are a lot simpler than we have made them. Start with being happy, go out there and take care of yourself so you can remain happy and spread the happy all around!

REFERENCES & GOOD STUFF

Perlmutter, David, and Kristin Loberg. *Grain Brain: The Surprising Truth about Wheat, Carbs, and Sugar--your Brain's Silent Killers.* New York: Little Brown &, 2013. Print.

Chek, Paul, How to Eat Move and Be Healthy: Your personalized 4 step guide to looking and feeling great from the inside out. San Diego, California: Paul Chek 2004.

Jackson, Bryan, The Book of Theta. Bryan Jackson, 2012.

https://www.centerpointe.com/holosync/

http://naplesfitnesscoaching.com/21-day-detox/

http://highperformancelivingonline.com/op/42-day-transformation

www.ingramcontent.com/pod-product-compliance
Lightning Source LLC
Chambersburg PA
CBHW060224290526
45789CB00003B/1405